the art
of living

lisa bentley

A POETIC JOURNEY AND RESOURCE FOR COMPULSIVE EATERS

ISBN: 978-1-7399419-5-6

Written and published by Lisa Bentley.
Cover design and illustrations by Lisa Bentley.

A CIP catalogue record for this book is available from The British Library.

www.lisabentley.co.uk

fear captured me
i'll help food said
and for decades
i listened

i would like to say a special
thank you to those beautiful
wise women around the world,
who helped me to see what
i never saw before.

and to L and H. always.

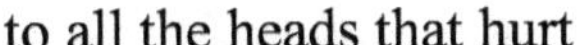
to all the heads that hurt

'That's another fine mess
you've gotten me into.'

Oliver Hardy

contents

'Do not worry that your life is turning upside down. How do you know the side you are used to is better than the one to come?' - Rumi

the
suffering

the art of living

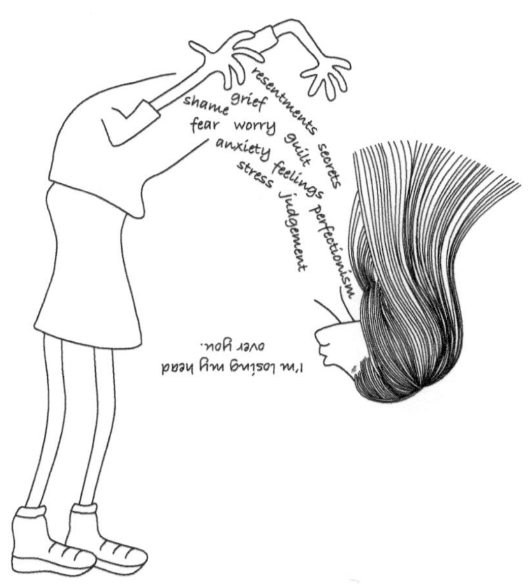
resentments secrets
grief
shame
fear worry guilt
anxiety feelings perfectionism
stress judgement
I'm losing my head
over you.

i want to pull myself together but
i'm not a pair of curtains

- off stage

my kItcHen
the wAr zone
where The battle
bEgins
my bathroom
in combat I am losing this fight
shE wins
        again.

- *I HATE ME*

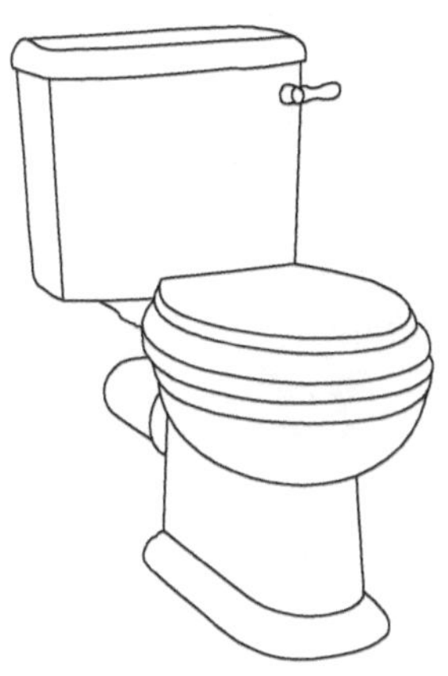

part my curtains
and the performance begins
special guests enter
one   by   one
the magician twirls and swirls
them around
teeth clap excitedly
ta da
the guests vanish
escaped through the trap door
encore, encore

and then there is
one
attire different than before
the audience is silenced
stilled
amazed
the curtains open
and the guests leave from where
they first came in

- the binge

as i curl over the table like a
shameful child
figuratively speaking i swallow
this glass of
arsenic i have been given
i metaphorically drink from
the cup of shame i have been
holding since
it started

- out of alignment

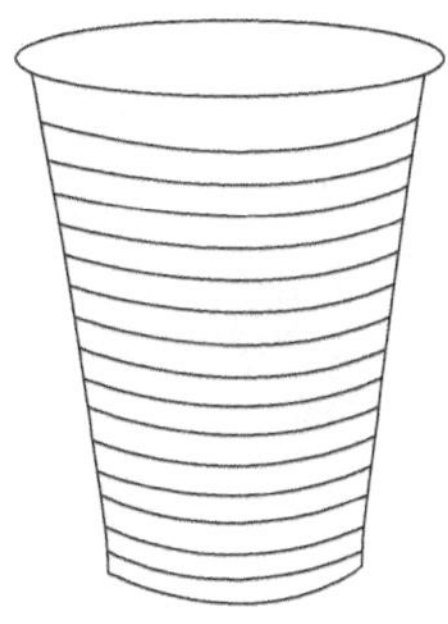

like ivy it attaches itself

- disordered eating

lisa bentley

some days i'm running to the
food some days i'm running

                 from it

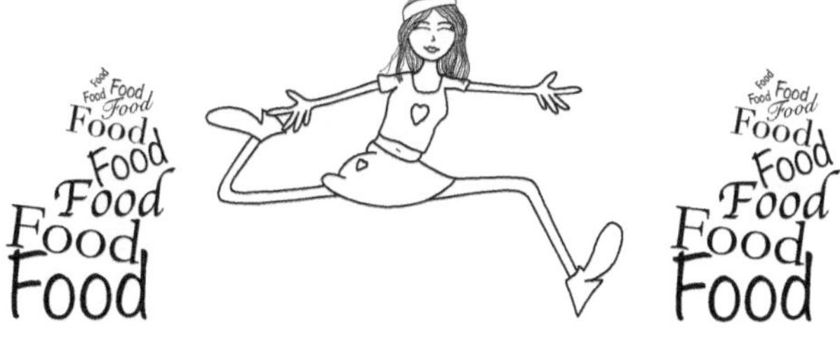

DIEt

- no cure

my tears are the glue that sticks
my hair to those cheeks
that once were as rosy
as the petals i watch
            falling
                from
                    the
                        bush
as the wind brushes by
and food numbs the emotions
that sizzle and spit inside of me
like hot fat that stings and burns
as it grasps around the breast of
the dead chicken that i cooked
and could then couldn't
            then should
                then shouldn't
                    then did
                        eat

- *powerlessness*

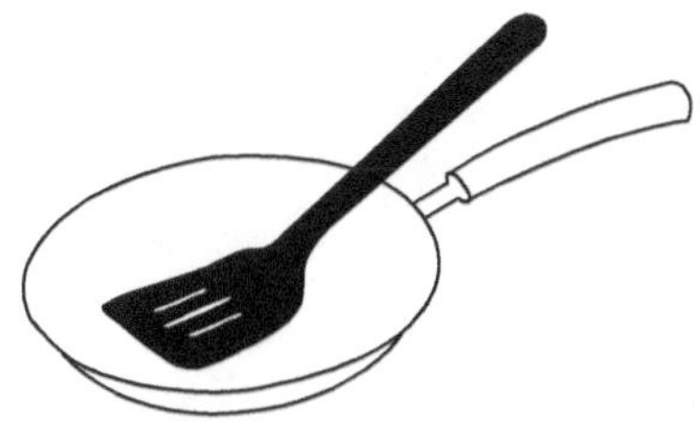

"Move over God, let me give you
a few tips."

- *Ego*

my self-will

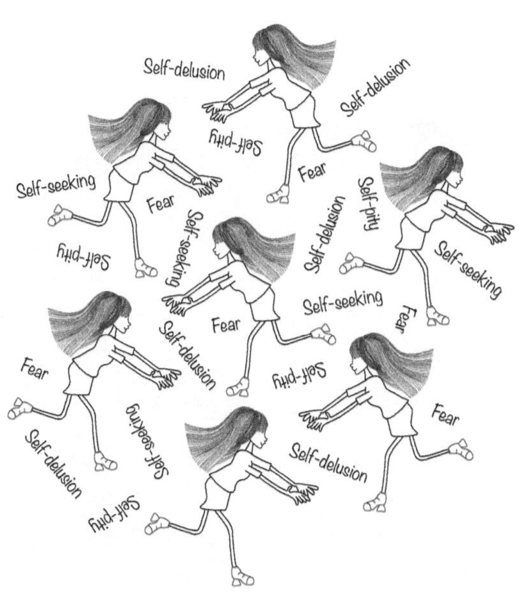

run riot

the truth is
you are always there
to help me through
you come
you comfort
you control
you lie.

- *food: friend or foe*

i can't control everything

- *including my hair*

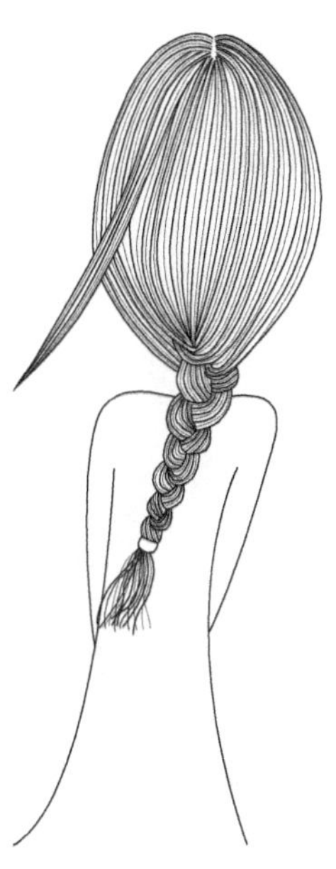

i can't control everything

my tongue dances and my teeth
        up
jump   and
              down
any exercise is better than none,
right?

- *excuses, excuses*

i hide it well?

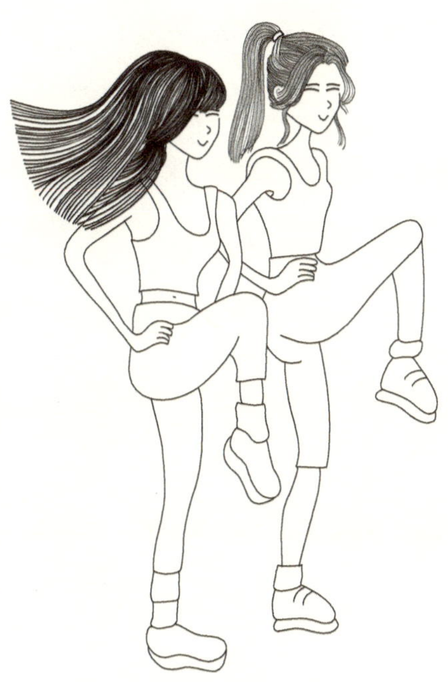

games i play:
      tug   of   war
       ladders
    &
snakes

dominoes
blind man's bluff
oranges and lemons

- the last one's dead!

if only everyone would do what i
wanted them to do then
everything would be
just fine

- irritable restless discontent

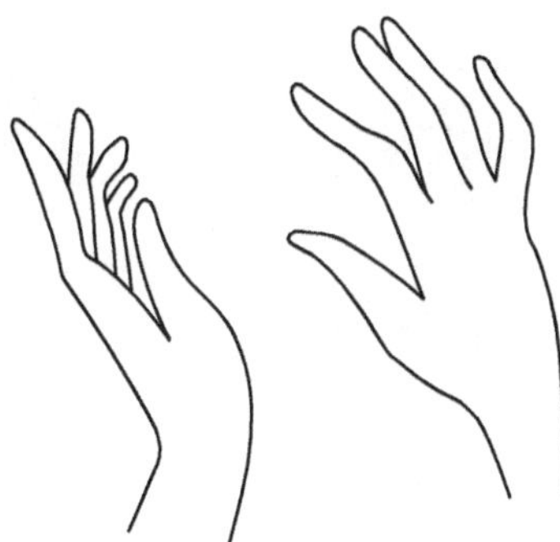

when life is out of alignment
        i

            mess

             u
               p

- off beam

control: the flip side of anxiety

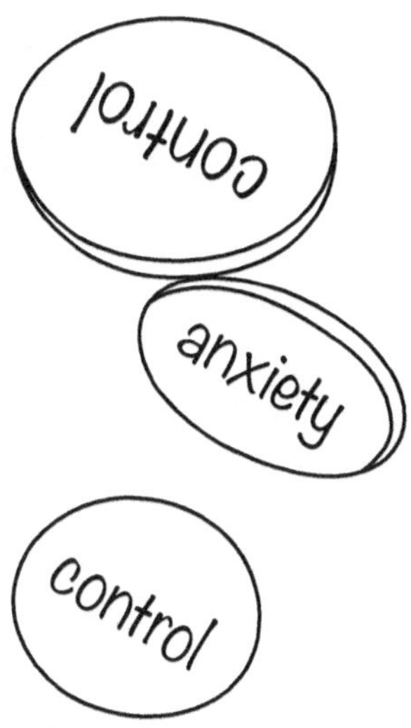

defective?

- or human

lisa bentley

love cuts deep

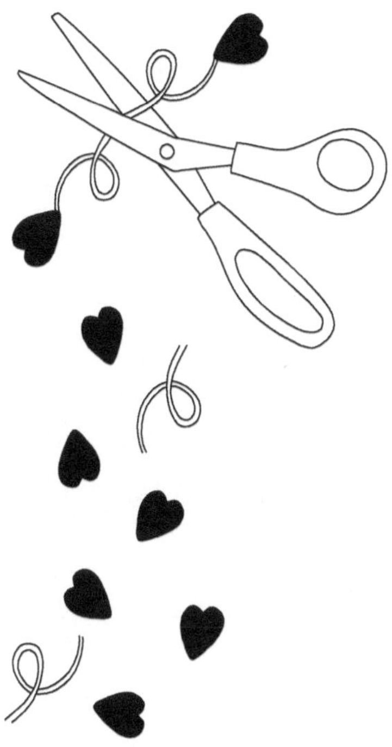

the primary *sauce* of my
suffering:

fear
people

- on my plate

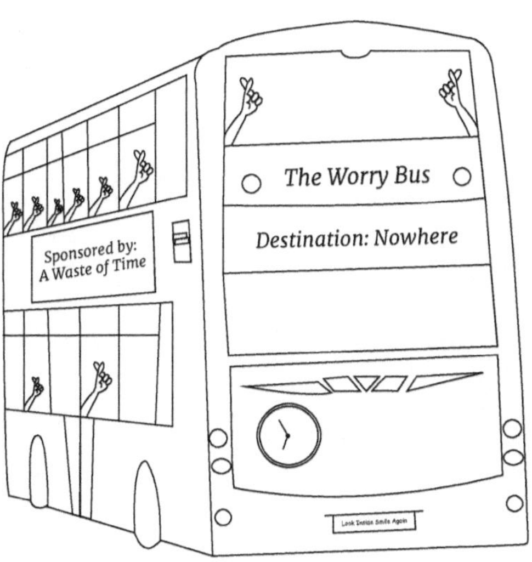
The Worry Bus
Destination: Nowhere
Sponsored by:
A Waste of Time
Look Inside Smile Again

sugar or breathing

- an easy choice?

when i keep chasing the feeling
eventually i run away with it

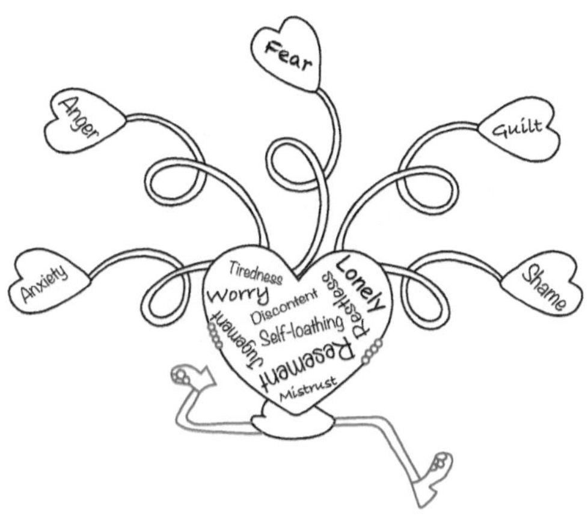

ice cream   i scream
   dread full   dreadful
      plaice   place

- *body v mind*

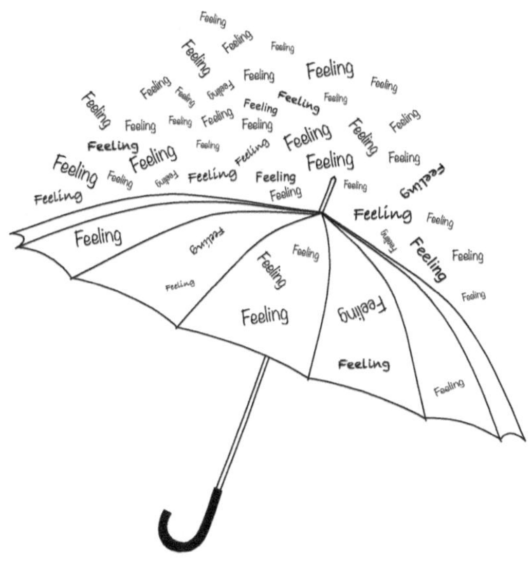

some days i'm flooded
with feelings

why do i do the same thing and
expect a different result?

- i'm insane

perfectionism: the perfect way to
prevent a perfect life

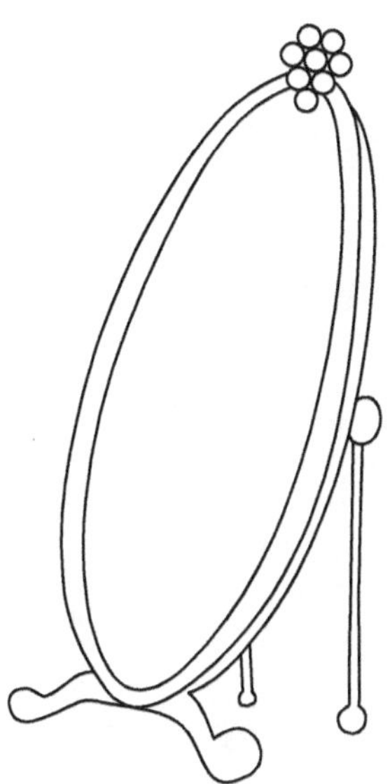

the
surrender

don't you think you've suffered
enough?

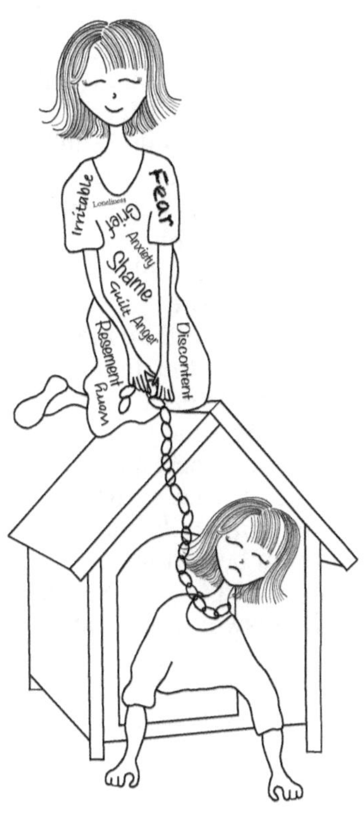

i'm standing in the dark with you
numbing out the pain
afraid that if the light comes on
my eyes will see disdain
my legs are still and heavy
mind and body don't entwine
what's wrong with me - i'm not content
i need to realign
you think everything is dandy
we're soul mates 'til the end
and standing in the dark with you
i consider you my friend
so do i stay or should i run?
your kindness keeps me here
but i'm scared of being on my own
you take aware this fear
i know i've been unkind to you
selfish to the core
in hope that you'll be mean enough
to push me out the door
standing in the dark i cry
not knowing what to do
trying to be honest and
authentic to what's true
contemplation tells me
i think i'm best to wait
surrender to a Higher Power
He will answer this debate.

- current conclusion

if i qUIt the debating team there's
a chance i'll find him

- a power greater than mine

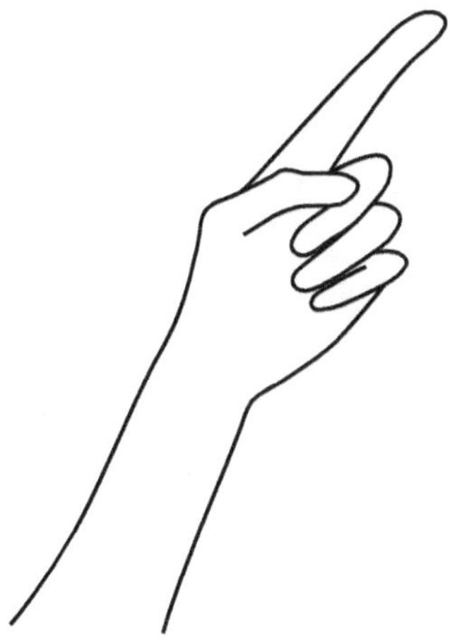

just because i didn't do it
yesterday doesn't mean i can't do
it today

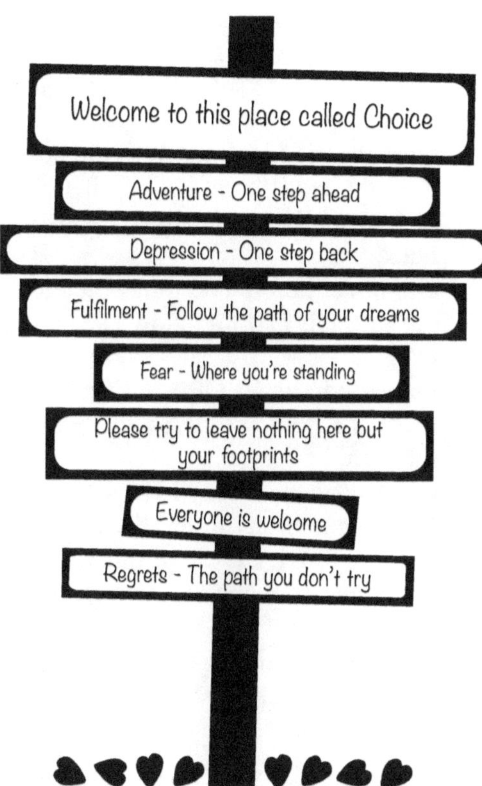

Welcome to this place called Choice
Adventure - One step ahead
Depression - One step back
Fulfilment - Follow the path of your dreams
Fear - Where you're standing
Please try to leave nothing here but your footprints
Everyone is welcome
Regrets - The path you don't try

out from my window
there is not much to see
just a red brick wall - it's GLARING at me!
i sit back in my chair
another day will pass by
this world that i live in, it feels like a LIE.
BUT
what if i tried looking from the next floor
it might be different behind that blue door?
so i take a DEEP breath and walk up to the
place
that never before had i the courage to face
out through *THIS* window i see more than a
wall
i see life in its GLORY - it's so beautiful!
there is a field with trees where a river runs
through
all this is here if only i knew
back home in my room, the wallCLOSESin
i've got to GET OUT of this mental dustbin!
that view from above was a glimmer of
HOPE
CHANGE IS the answer
i untie the thick rope.

- the shift

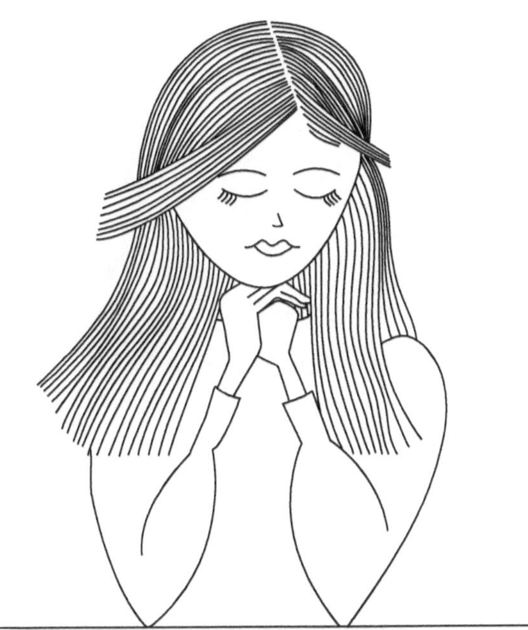

because nothing else worked

your house is so neat and tidy
they say. i SMiLE POLiTELY

so why can't my FEELiNGS be
too?

faith carries less weight

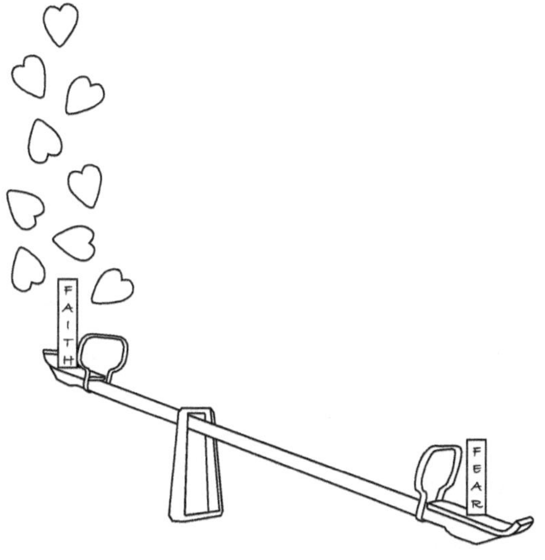

if i'm not going to feel
uncomfortable then i'm never
going to make a change

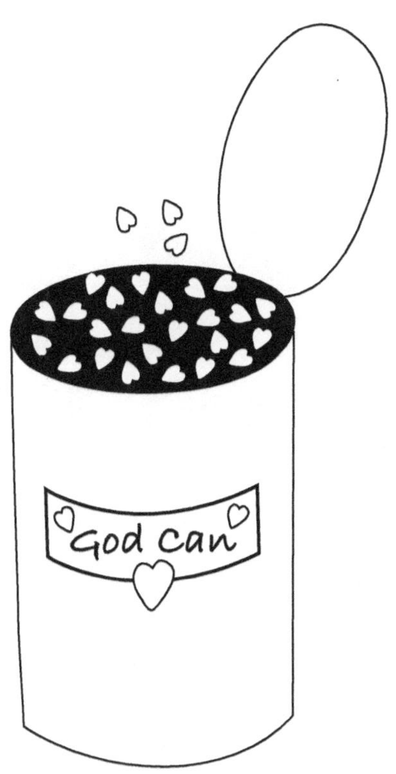

God can

don't stack the negative

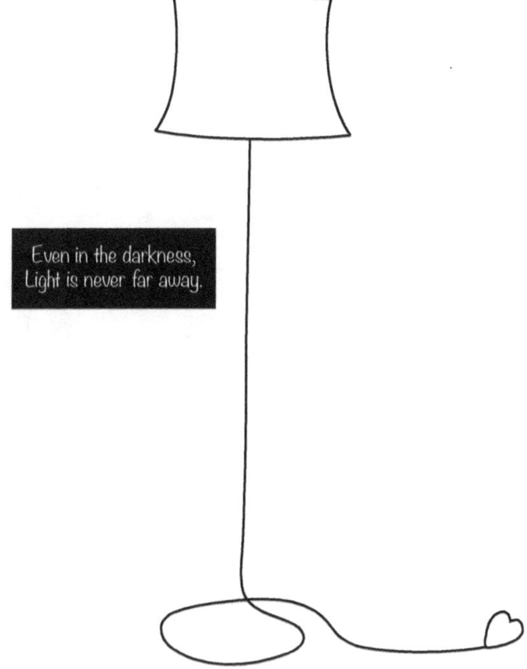
Even in the darkness,
Light is never far away.

when my shovel won't dig any
further

- *rock bottom*

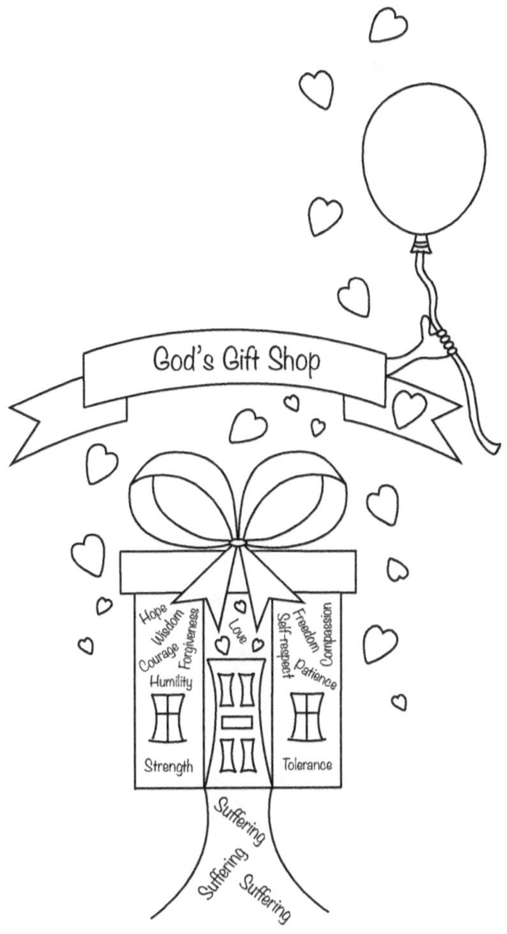
God's Gift Shop
Hope
Wisdom
Courage
Forgiveness
Humility
Love
Freedom
Self-respect
Compassion
Patience
Strength
Tolerance
Suffering
Suffering
Suffering

a fish in water doesn't know it's
surrounded by water until it's
taken out

- *toxic pond*

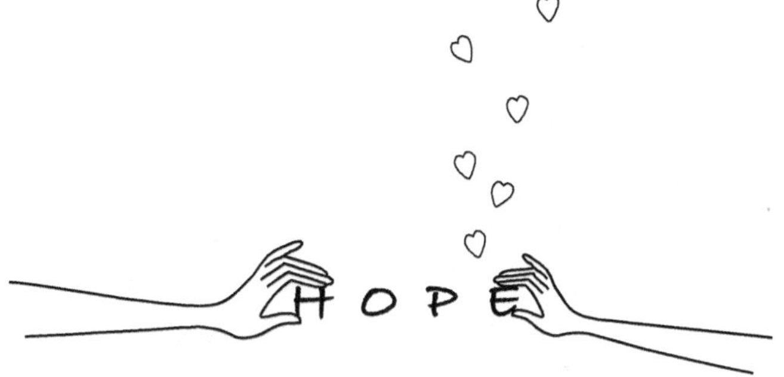
HOPE

the
solution

the art of living

62

step into the colour

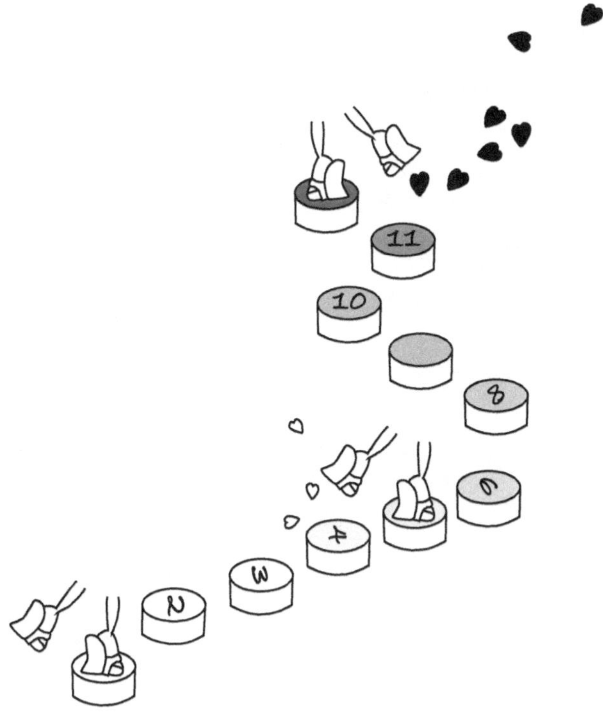

desperation is a gift

getting clean

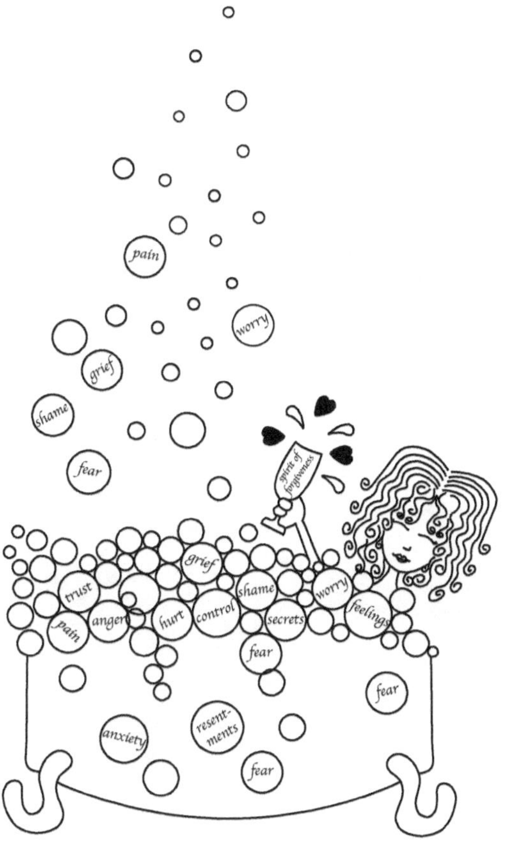

i'm learning that *emotional* states
dominate me. *not food*

lisa bentley

should i staple my mouth or heart
first?

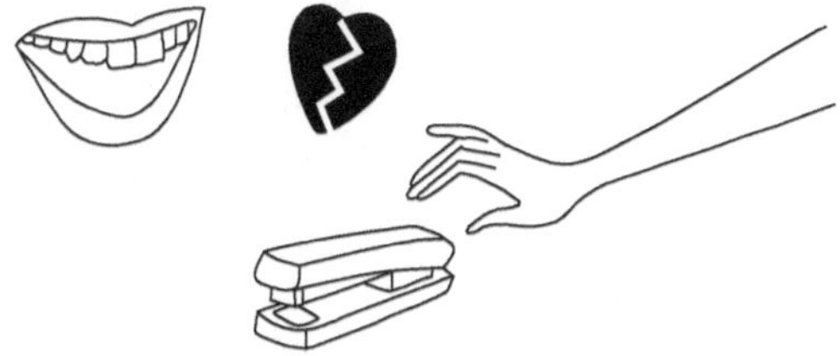

forgiveness is just a suggestion
like the rip cord when jumping
out of a plane is just a suggestion

emotional baggage has legs

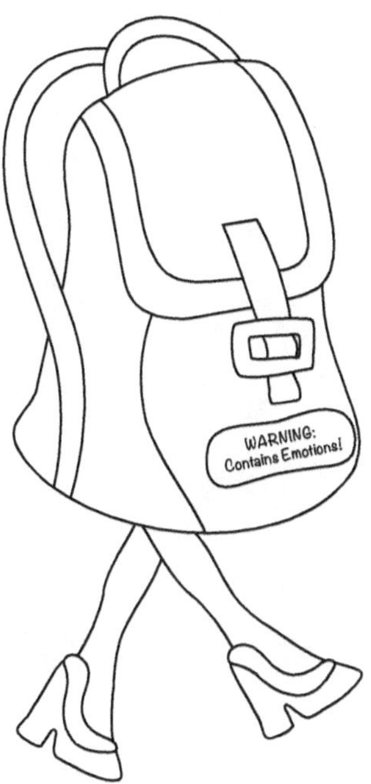

emotional baggage has legs

any place i do i do every place

don't fence yourself in

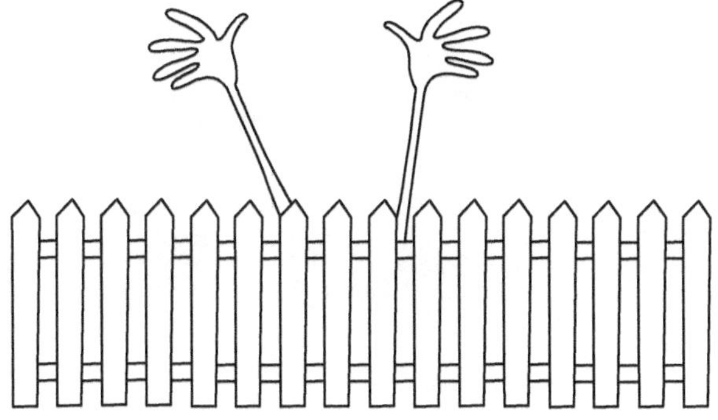

what lies do you tell yourself?

kindness makes other hearts sing

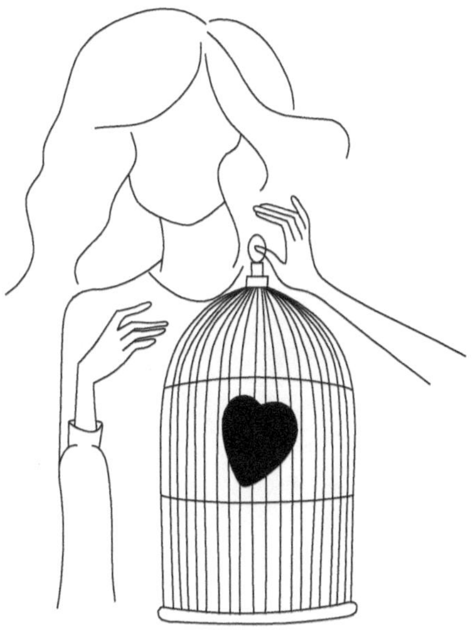

reduce conflict by planning

- keep it simple

hang up the gloves

- let go

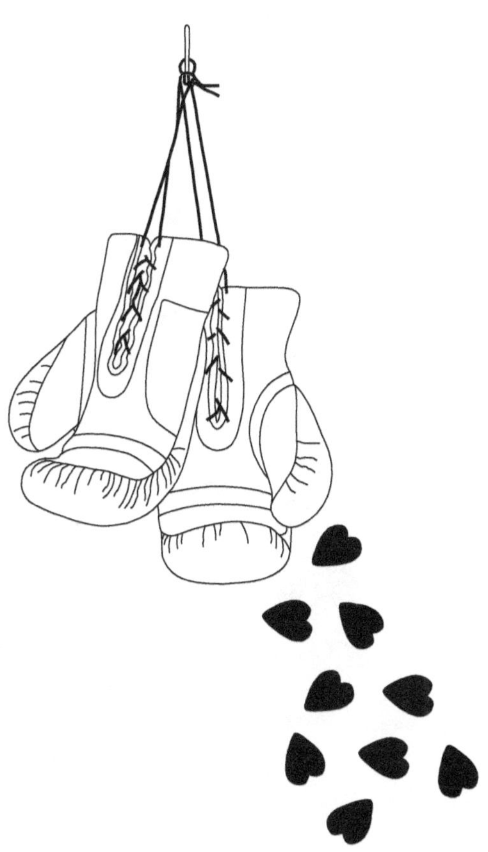

my expectations are the cause of
my pain

- *not the person nor the food*

we all own an empty jar. it's our
choice what we fill it with.

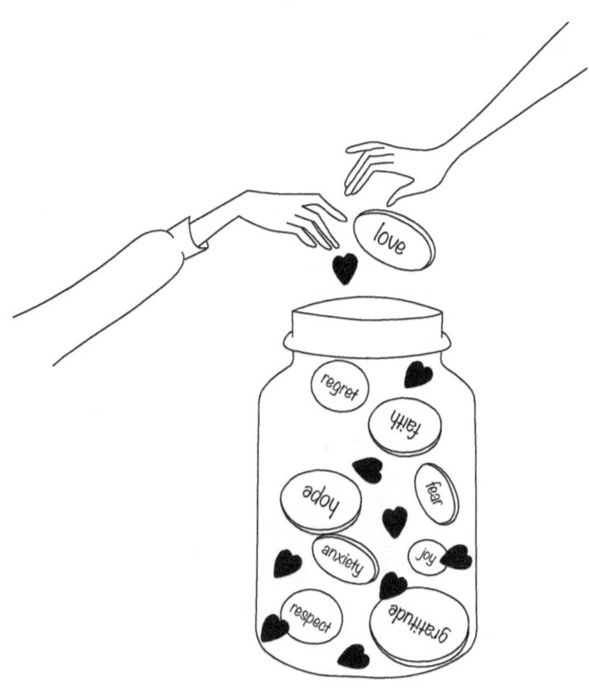

love yourself

- it's your duty

self-love is nothing to feel
ashamed of

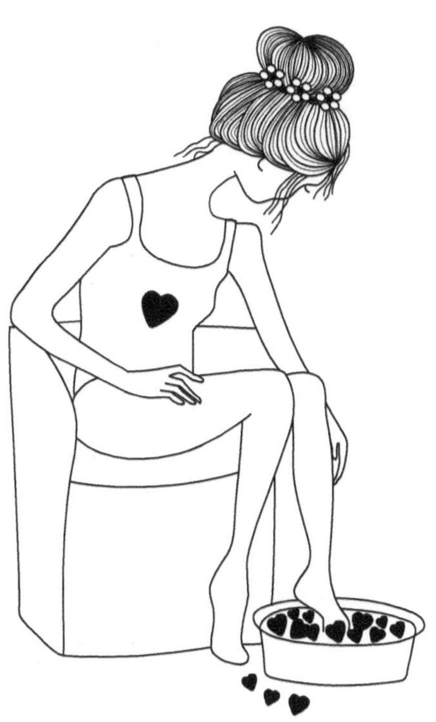

no one's too old to create a new
future

- *you're worth it*

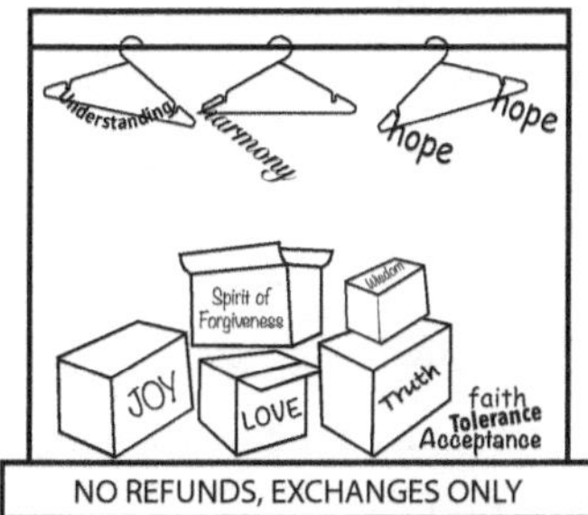

RETURNS DEPT
Understanding
Harmony
hope
Hope
Spirit of Forgiveness
Wisdom
JOY
LOVE
Truth
faith
Tolerance
Acceptance
NO REFUNDS, EXCHANGES ONLY

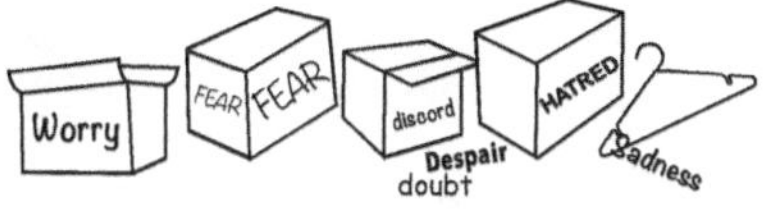

Worry
FEAR
FEAR
discord
Despair
doubt
HATRED
Sadness

go easy on yourself

it's time to gently unpack it all

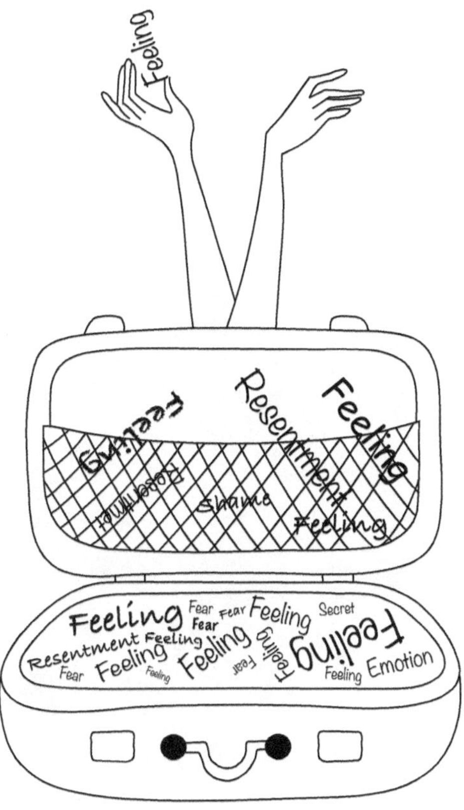

rather than stuffing my face i'm
facing my stuff

- acceptance

stop hanging on to those negative
thoughts

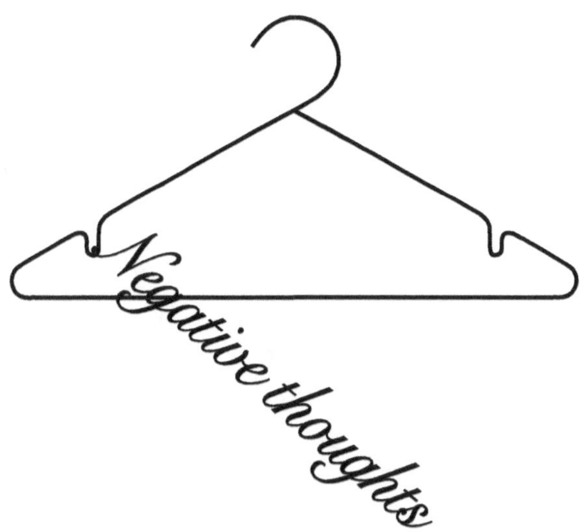

stoves

sewers

- *my analogy of life*

don't get tangled up in knots

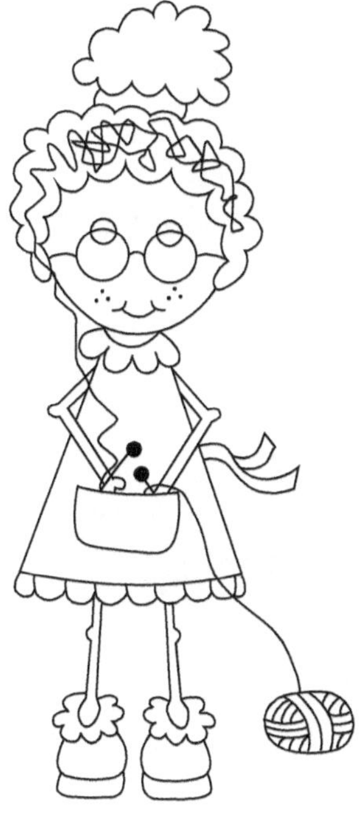

Forgive Everyone And Recover

- fear

recalibrate regularly

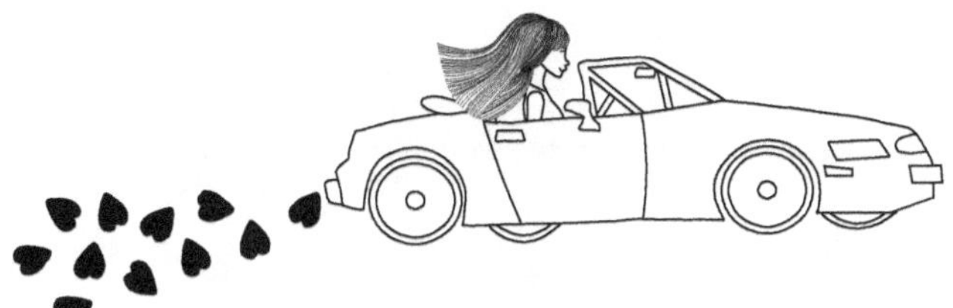

i need to sip lemon-aid instead of
chewing on beef

- *with myself*

lisa bentley

don't salt that thought

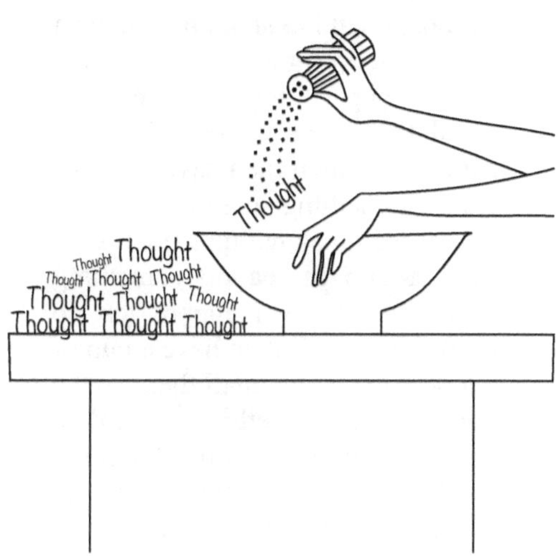

do something small then have a cup
of tea do something small then have
a cup of tea do something small
then have a cup of tea do something
small then have a cup of tea do
something small then have a cup of
tea do something small then have a
cup of tea do something small then
have a cup of tea do something
small then have a cup of tea do
something small then have a cup of
tea do something small then have a
cup of tea do something small then
have a cup of tea do something
small then have a cup of tea do
something small then have a cup of
tea do something small then have a
cup of tea do something small then
have a cup of tea do something
small then have a cup of tea do
something small then have a cup of
tea do something small then have a
cup of tea do something small then
have a cup of tea do something
small then have a cup of tea do
something small then have a cup of
tea do something small then have a
cup of tea do something small then
have a cup of tea do something
small then have a cup of tea do
something small then have a cup of
tea do something small then have a
cup of tea do something small then
have a cup of tea do something
small then have a cup of tea do
something small then have a cup of

tea do something small then have a
cup of tea do something small then
have a cup of tea do something
small then have a cup of tea do
something small then have a cup of
tea do something small then have a
cup of tea do something small then
have a cup of tea do something
small then have a cup of tea do
something small then have a cup of
tea do something small then have a
cup of tea do something small then
have a cup of tea do something
small then have a cup of tea do
something small then have a cup of
tea do something small then have a
cup of tea do something small then
have a cup of tea do something
small then have a cup of tea do
something small then have a cup of
tea do something small then have a
cup of tea do something small then
have a cup of tea do something
small then have a cup of tea do
something small then have a cup of
tea do something small then have a
cup of tea do something small then
have a cup of tea do something
small then have a cup of tea do
something small then have a cup of
tea do something small then have a
cup of tea do something small then
have a cup of tea.

- *thirsty work*

there's never going to be a time
when there aren't feelings

- *as long as i'm breathing*

make time for you

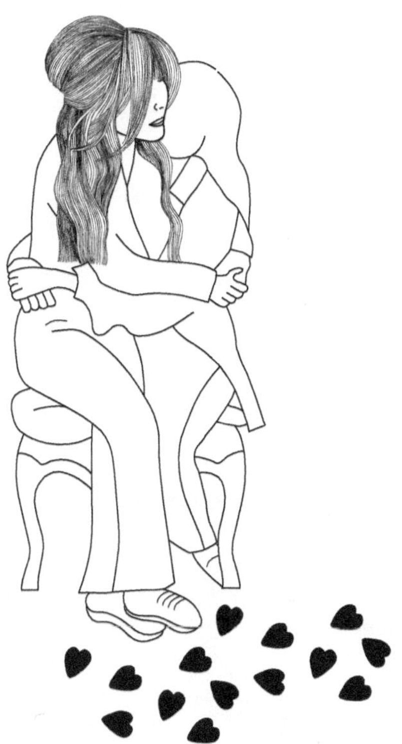

we might love cheese. it's a
shame, but it's not the end of the
world. the sun will still rise.

- hopeFUL

nurture your inner child

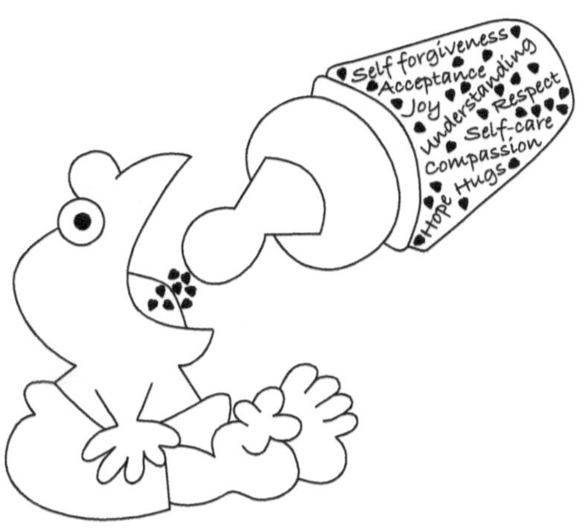

pay the farmer not the chemist

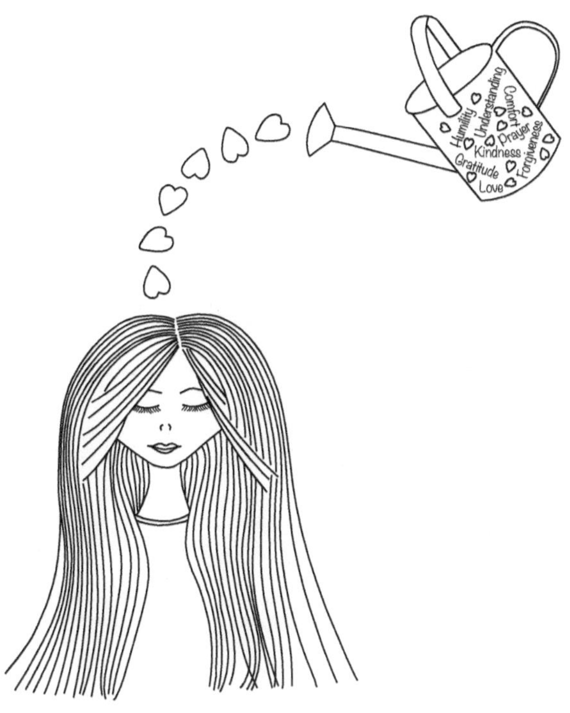

Humility
Understanding
Comfort
Prayer
Kindness
Forgiveness
Gratitude
Love

fear is physical – courage feels
different

don't let anyone be the Director
of your life

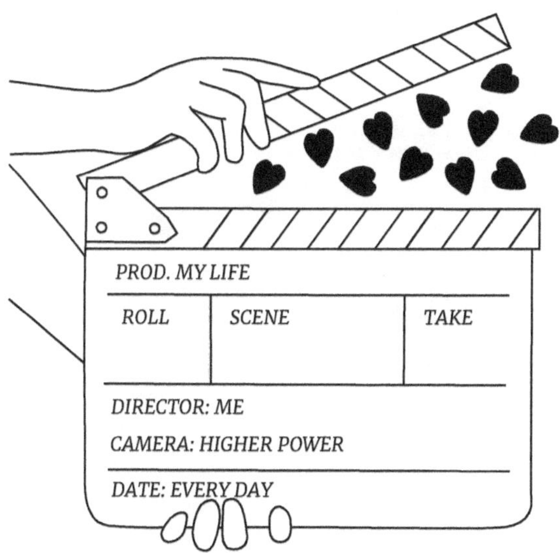

how may we grow from our
actions?

- *cultivation*

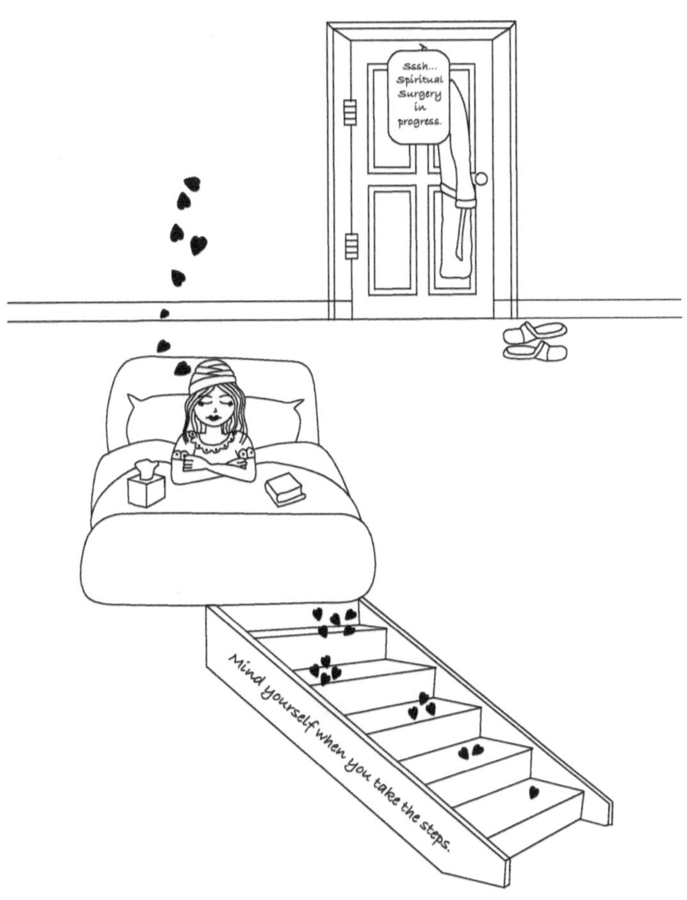
Sssh...
Spiritual
Surgery
in
progress.
Mind yourself when you take the steps.

three meals a day, life in between

when one's too many and ten
isn't enough

*- based on the quote by Brendan
Behan and in homage to The Big
Book of AA*

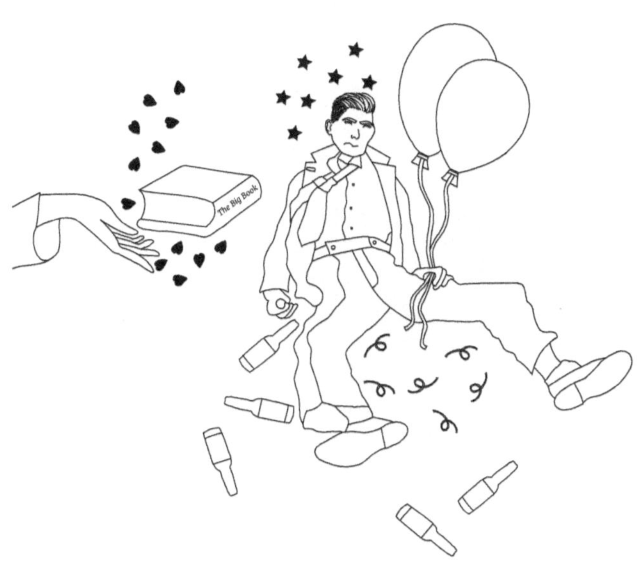

WAIT
Why Am I Talking?

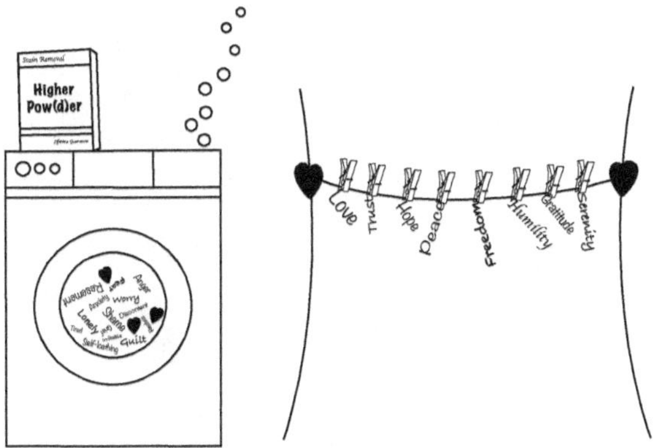

Stain Removal
Higher Pow(d)er
lifetime guarantee
Resentment
Fear
Anger
Anxiety
Worry
Lonely
Shame
Discomfort
Tired
Self-loathing
Guilt
Love
Trust
Hope
Peace
Freedom
Humility
Gratitude
Serenity

a camel starts their day on its
knees
it ends on them too

- *act like a camel*

don't measure self-worth by
these scales

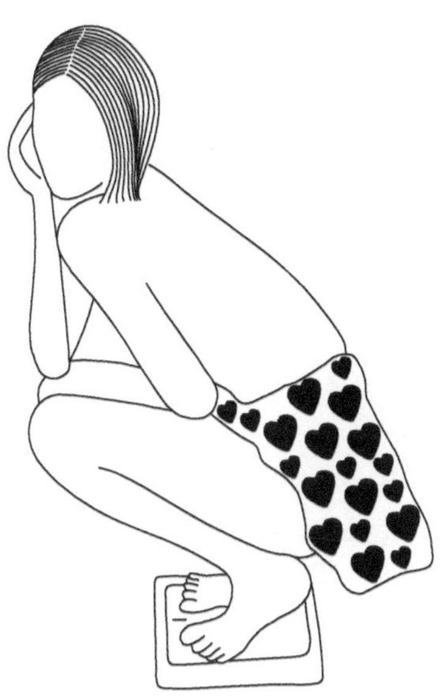

see
saws
rollercoasters
swings
    rOundabOuts
obstacle courses
C
L
I
M
B
I
N
G
    frames

- life

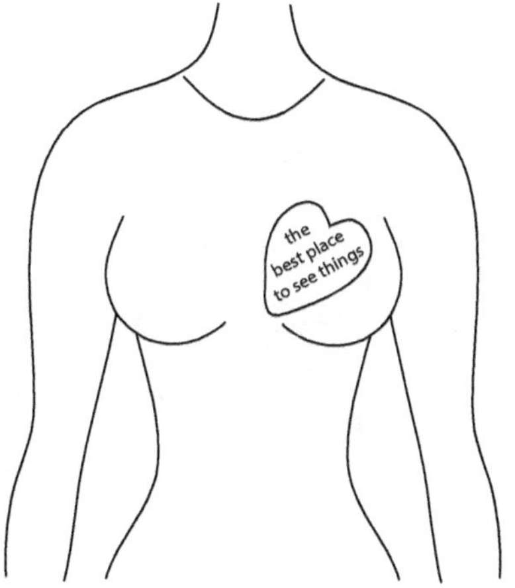
the
best place
to see things

the more i look up the harder it
becomes to look down

lisa bentley

i'm putting pride in my pocket

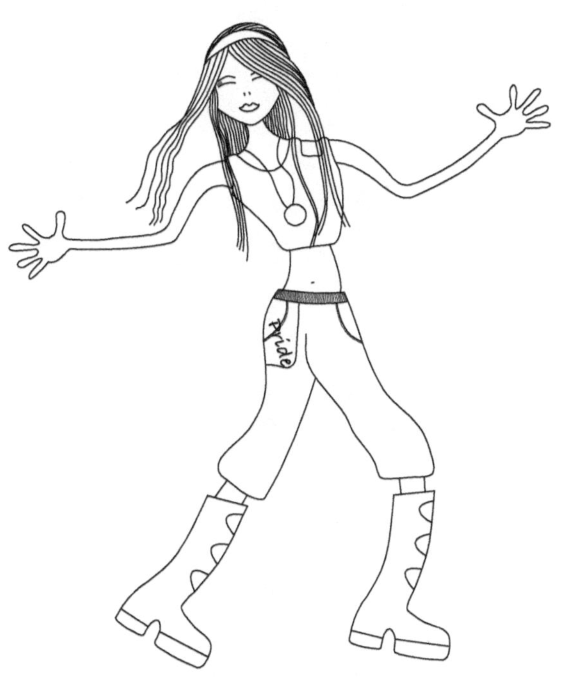

is it a thought or a feeling?
sometimes we think we are
feeling something when in fact
it's just a thought

you are enough

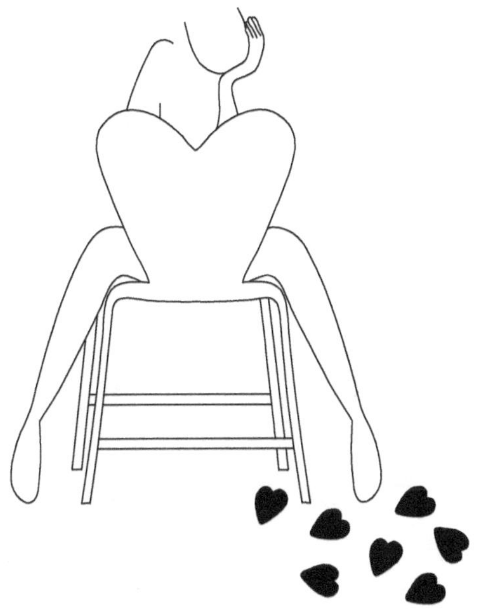

how may i grow from pausing

be brave enough to do the things
that fill your heart with joy

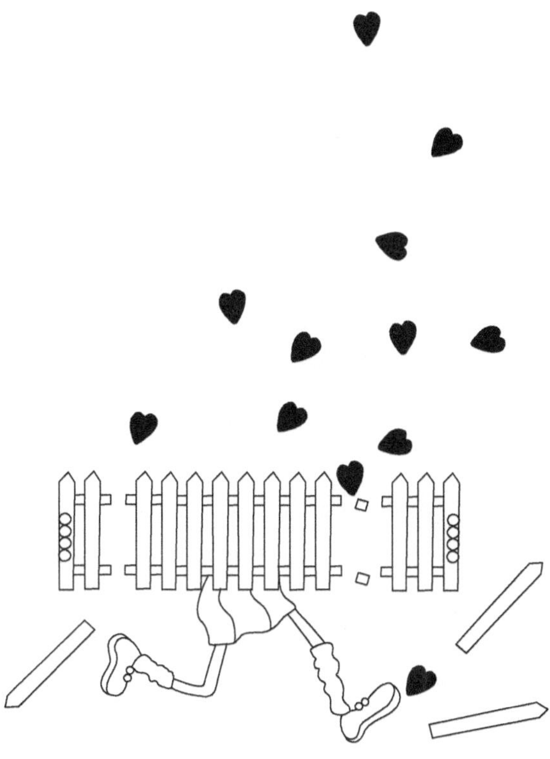

bless them change me

what are my feet doing?

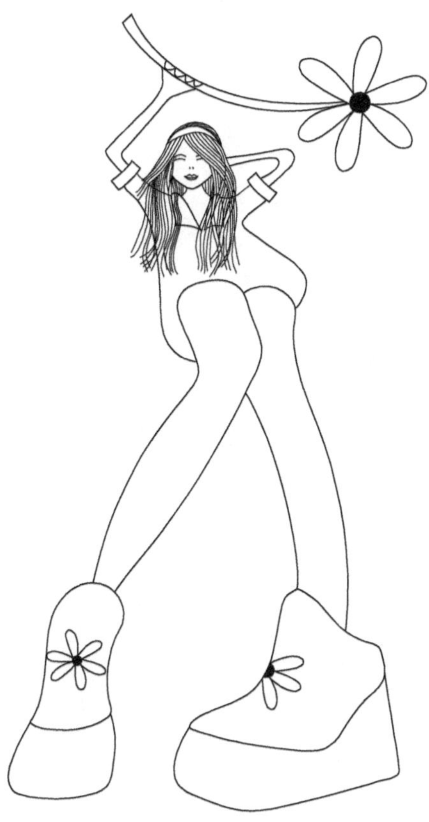

does it need to be said
does it need to be said now
does it need to be said by me

- less is more

come home to yourself

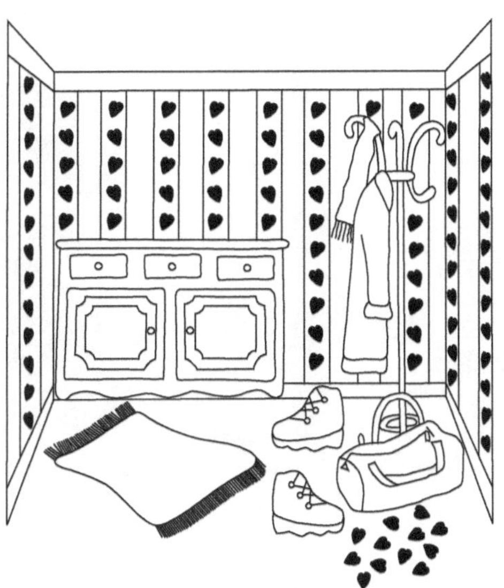

like a seed i'm stronger than i
think

i wish i could vacuum up my character defects

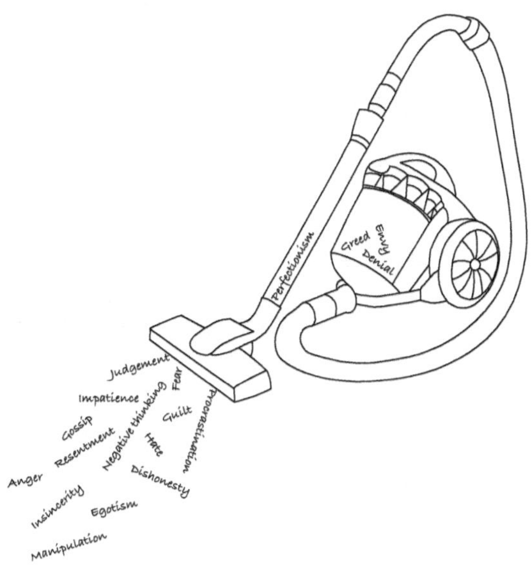

a flower needs dirt in order to
grOW

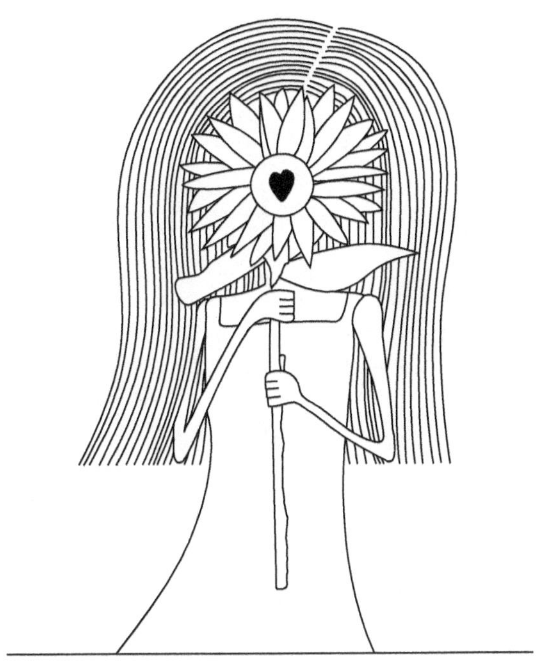

when i procrastinate my life
becomes unmanageable

reach out to others

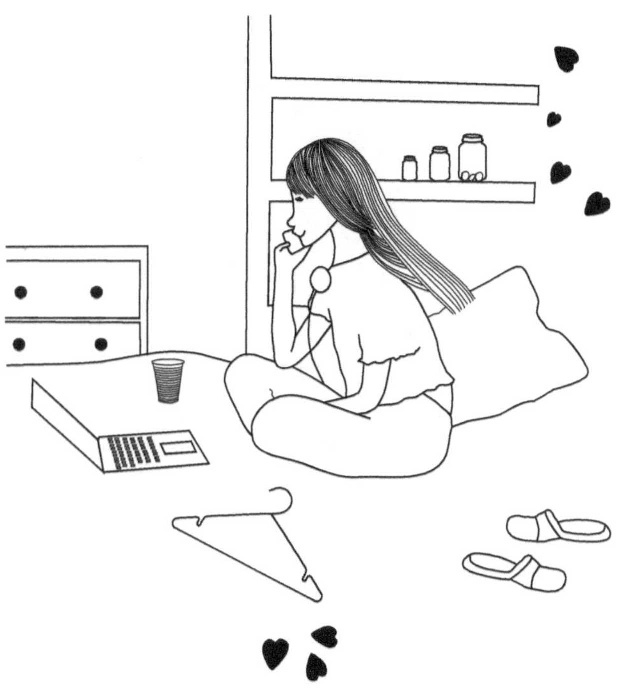

these days, when i fall, i get up a
lot quicker

reach out again and again and
again

- strength in numbers

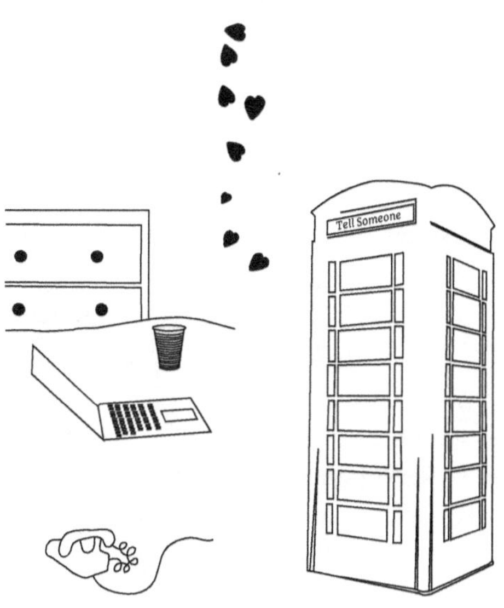

you smiled and would laugh
– i thought you really cared
serving up plates of food
          i ate but i was scared
you took me in when i was weak;
emotionally i was broke

BUT DOES THAT REALLY JUSTIFY
HARSH WORDS THAT YOU ONCE
SPOKE?

you pretended you were
          someone else
when people rang the phone
you told me:
          'YOU ARE NOT TO WORK!'
                    – this cut me to the bone

controlling every move i made and
judging every day
inside my head i screamed and sobbed:
'PLEASE JUST GO AWAY!'

you told me, 'I AM NOT TO MOVE'
– were you afraid for me?
or was it your own selfishness
          – this I didn't see

but as the years passed me by
and i got to know you well
sometimes i'd sit and wonder why
YOU MADE MY LIFE SUCH HELL

NEVER ONCE did you ask
        how and if i cope
if you had
you might have seen me
        walking a tightrope
turning to the food i ate,
suppressing my own grief
covering up the anguish that was living
underneath
i internalise why you chose
        to poke around my house
why didn't i confront you?
– I'M A LEO not a mouse!

inside my mind is screaming:
'YOU STOLE MY TRUST IN YOU!'
and i question if you sleep at night
knowing what you do

The Big Book i have read aloud
i now live for just today

i surrender
i am powerless
i contemplate
i pray

FORGIVENESS is the only way i've
learned will heal my pain
and fencing you outside of me will help
to keep me sane.

- the thief

just for today i'm not dancing
around controlled use

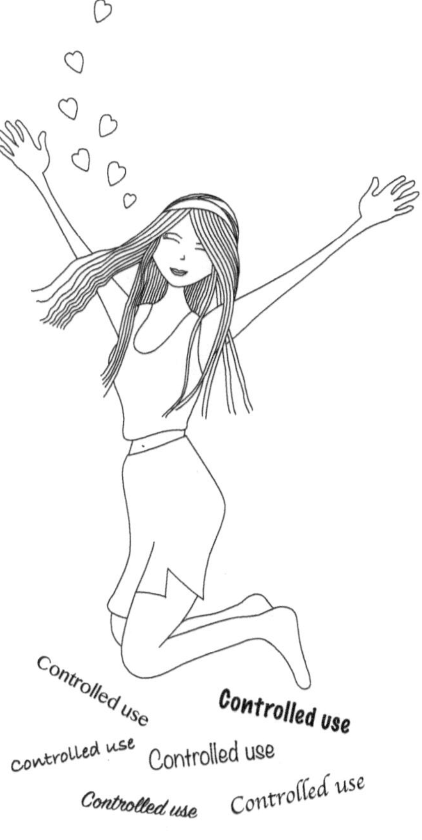

my behavior tells me what i believe

lisa bentley

iron out our differences
sweep away our prejudices

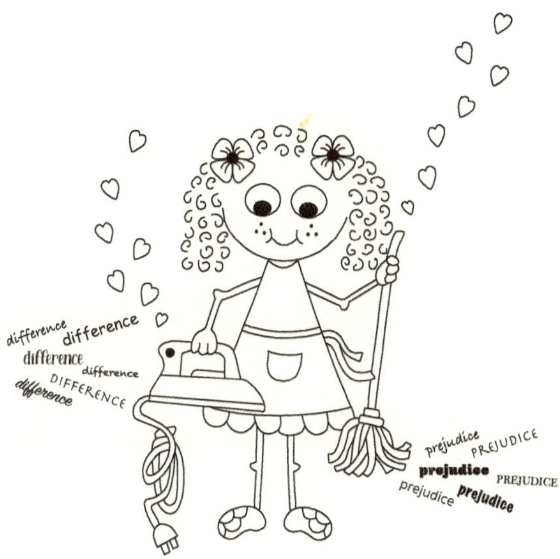

food wasn't my problem
it was my solution

lisa bentley

freedom from the bondage of self

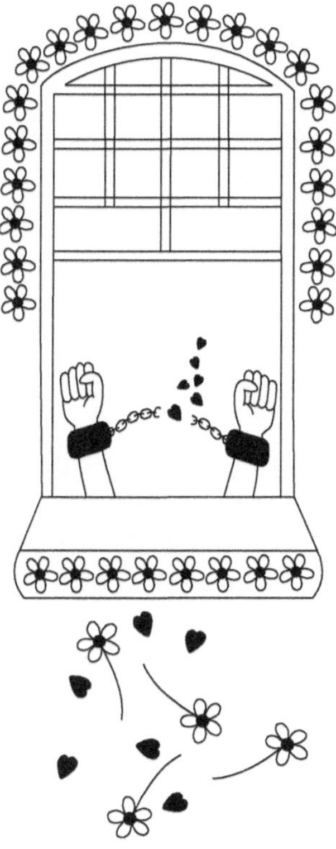

what am i hungry for?

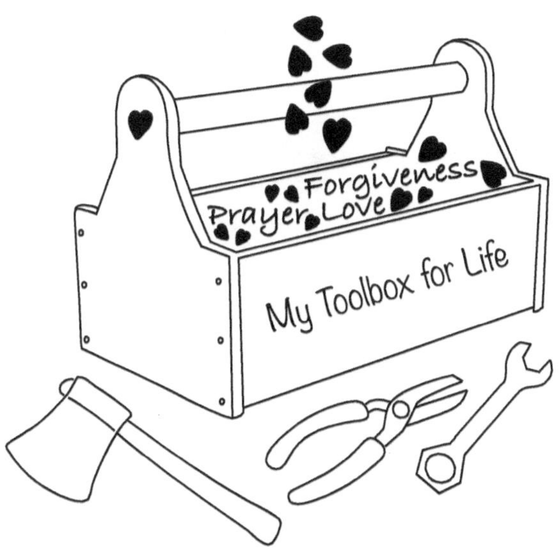

Forgiveness
Prayer Love
My Toolbox for Life

the art of living

the
service

the art of living

share the love

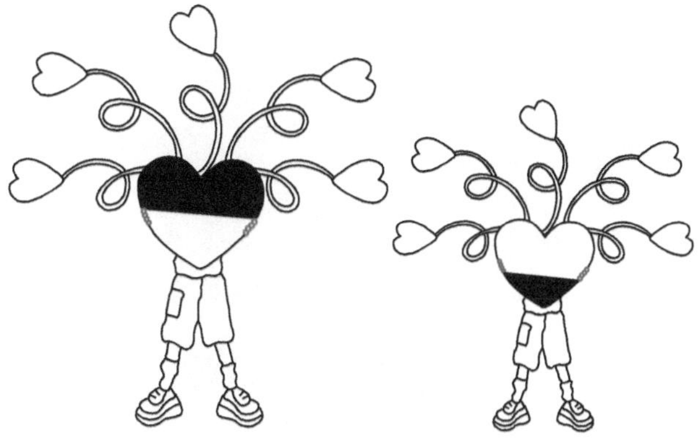

helping others is a little bit of
insurance against myself for not
slipping

lisa bentley

I   self-love
O   love others
U   u will heal

- paycheck

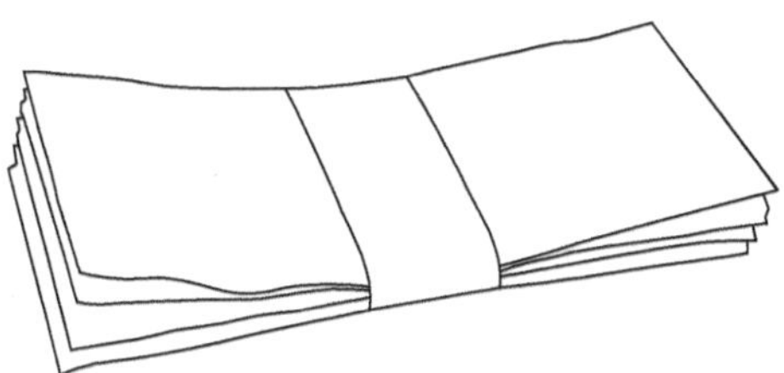

the wound is there, but there's
peace in my heart.

serve the world every day

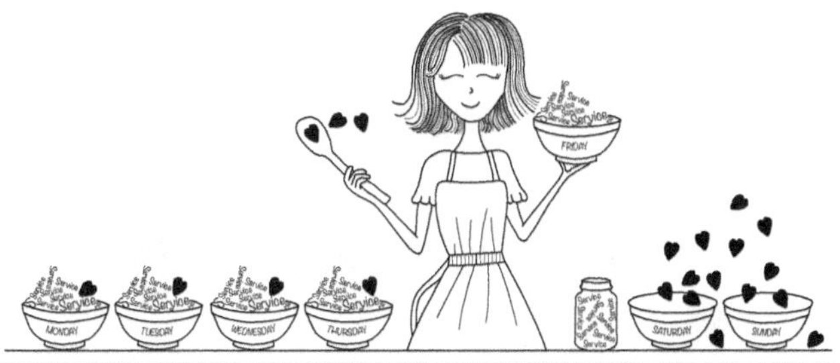

whether you say you can or say
you can't, you're right

- *stay humble*

for today my obsession is lifted

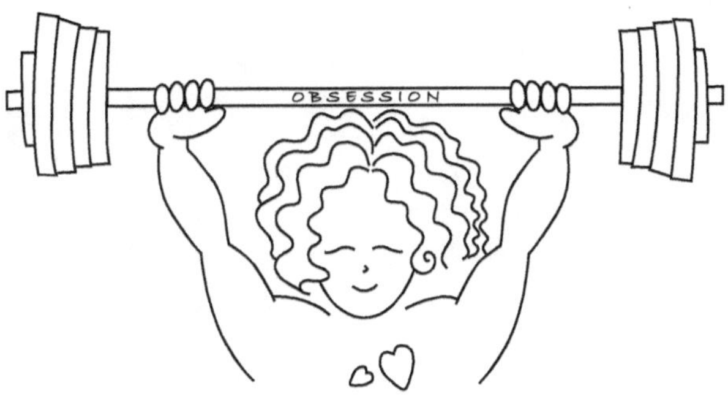

u and i aren't so difference
we are from the same source

- *my alphabet*

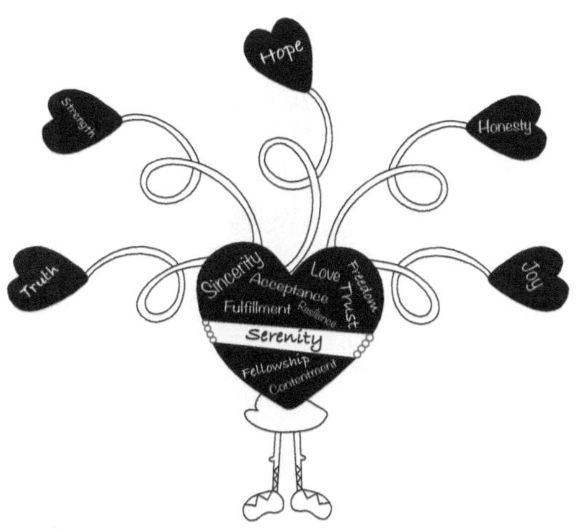

Hope
Strength
Honesty
Truth
Joy
Sincerity
Love
Freedom
Acceptance
Trust
Fulfillment
Resilience
Serenity
Fellowship
Contentment

the sea isn't scared to move and
make w a v e s
and the wind often alters the way
it   b eh a ve s
the moon has no choice but to
come OUT at night
and the sun is designed to stay
hot and shine bright

- *you: a special creation*

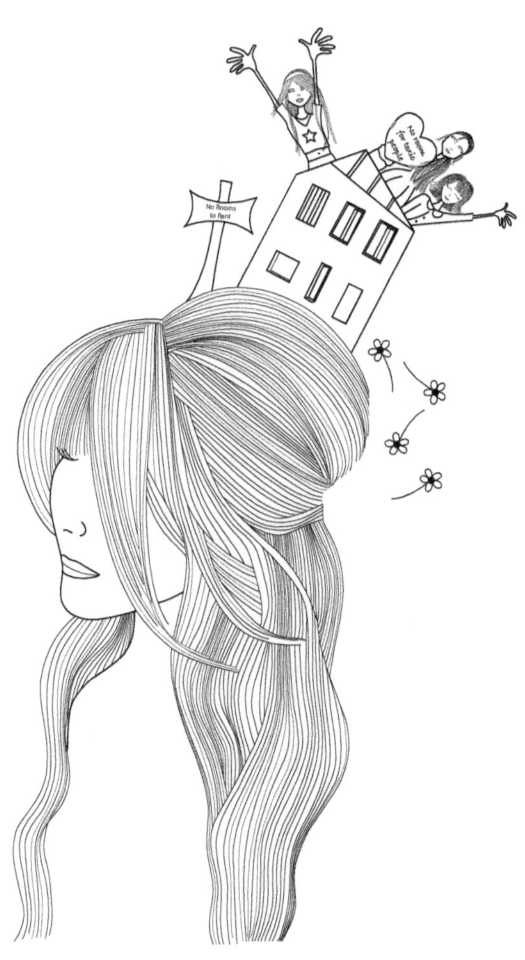
No Rooms
to Rent

no longer is my mind ransacked
by
anguish
and
fear
and
hurt
and
pain
no longer am i dismantled and
living in p i e c e s
by being of service my hole can
be whole

- a receipt

i'm using the tongue in my shoe
not the one in my mouth

- *daily focus*

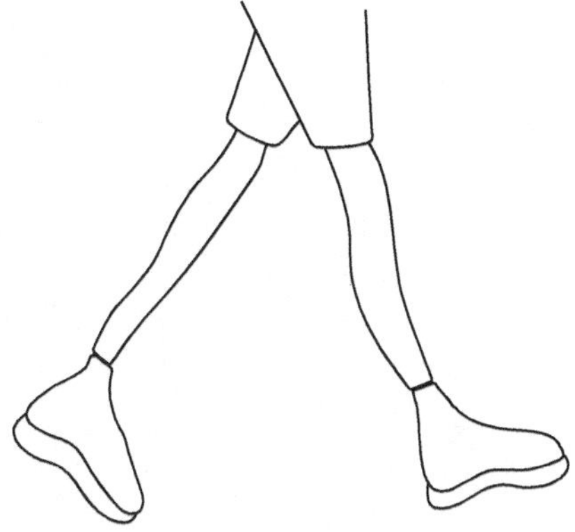

i haven't changed but how i do
things has changed

carry the message not the mess

- 12 step advice

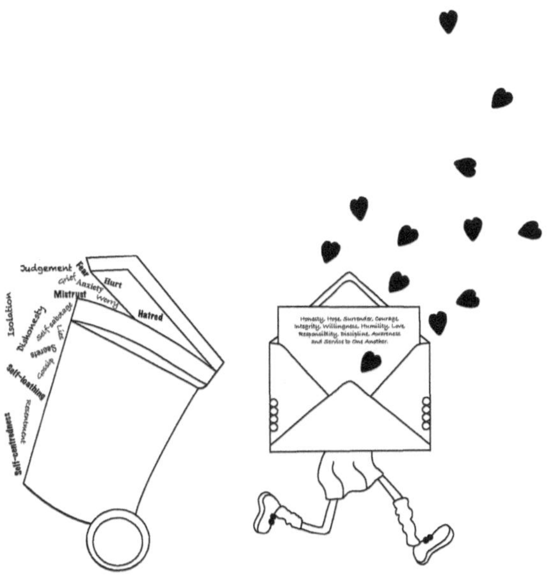

when i fall i get up a lot quicker

when i fall i get up a lot quicker

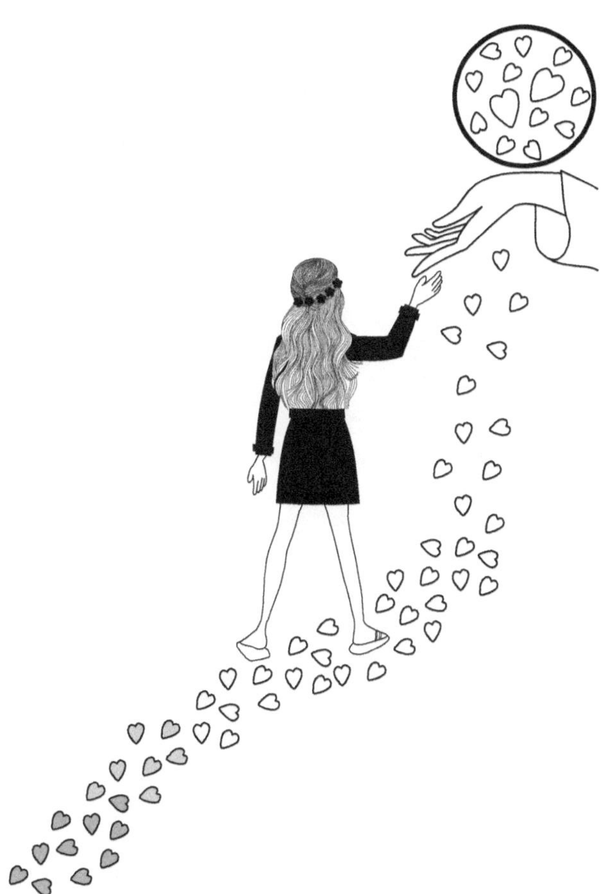

piece by piece i'm finding peace

- *one day at a time*

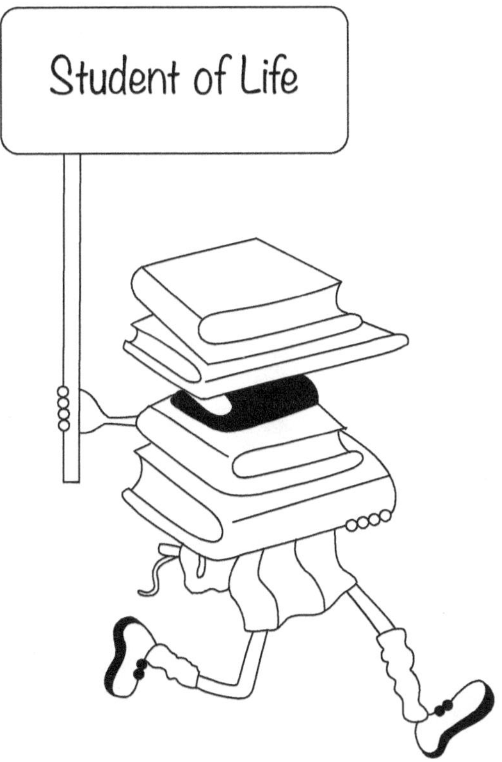
Student of Life

reflections

lisa bentley

reflections

reflections

lisa bentley

reflections

reflections

lisa bentley

reflections

167

reflections

lisa bentley

reflections

reflections

lisa bentley

reflections

reflections

lisa bentley

reflections

reflections

lisa bentley

reflections

reflections

lisa bentley

reflections

reflections

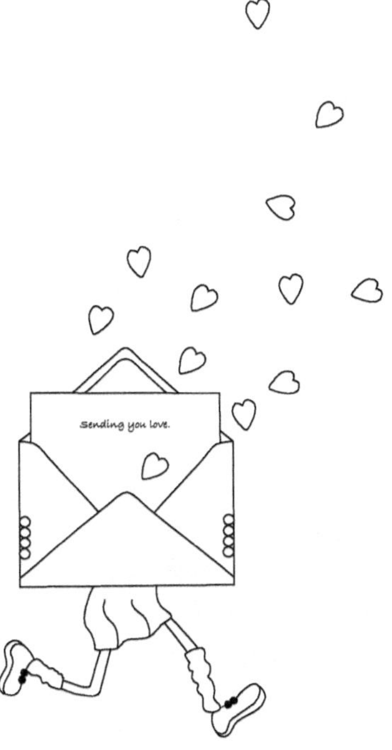
Sending you love.

i am sorry for the way i blamed you, shamed
you, craved you, resented you, all because
i wanted both you and me to be ok. back
then, in the grips of my disease, i was
living a life by my standards; i
wasn't considering you at all,
even though i thought i was.
i wanted you to be ok,
but i wanted me to
be ok more. i
manipulated
you; fear
is no
excuse.
i judged and had expectations that were
not fair. i am sorry for that. i was selfish,
self-seeking and i'm deeply sorry.
i love you and i'm learning.
i'm learning to let go.
i'm learning so
much and
for today
i know
better.

- an amends to my body

there are many tools to recovery;
creativity became one of mine.
from the pen to the paper,
from the keyboard to the screen,
it is there that i found connection and hope,
fellowship and wisdom, freedom and joy,
and a Power greater than mine.
i will forever be indebted.

by letting go i got strong
and by pausing i grew wise.
may my words and art serve you
one day at a time.

- with love x

www.ingramcontent.com/pod-product-compliance
Lightning Source LLC
Chambersburg PA
CBHW022052050726
47591CB00002B/501